Dash Diet Recipes

Lower your Blood Pressure and Increase your Energy with Easy Mouth-watering Recipes

Chloe Brockton

no scenarios in which the publisher or the original author of this work can be in any fashion deemed liable for any hardship or damages that may befall them after undertaking information described herein.

Additionally, the information in the following pages is intended only for informational purposes and should thus be thought of as universal. As befitting its nature, it is presented without assurance regarding its prolonged validity or interim quality. Trademarks that are mentioned are done without written consent and can in no way be considered an endorsement from the trademark holder.

Table of Contents

INTRODUCTION.. 7

DASH DIET RECIPES 9

Greek Yogurt Oat Pancakes.. 10

Breakfast Bread Pudding.. 11

Apple Pancakes 13

Avocado Nori Rolls 14

Perfect Granola 16

Spinach Muffins... 18

Healthy Breakfast Cookies... 19

Mediterranean Toast... 21

No-Bake Breakfast Granola Bars 22

Strawberry Sandwich... 24

Salmon Topper Stuffed Avocados.............................. 25

Creamy Chicken Breast.. 26

Chicken, Bamboo, and Chestnuts Mix 27

Sunshine Wrap 29

Pesto and Mozzarella Stuffed Portobello Mushroom Caps....... 31

Creamy Pumpkin Pasta.. 32

Avocado Cup with Egg... 34

Chicken Vegetable Soup 35

Salsa Chicken... 37

Sweet Potato Soup 39

Pear, Turkey and Cheese Sandwich 40

Turkey Meatloaf 41

Pesto Shrimp Pasta 43

Hot Chicken Wings 45

Spinach-Orzo Salad with Chickpeas 46

Black Bean and Sweet Potato Rice Bowls 48

Paprika Lamb Chops 50

Zucchini Beef Sauté with Coriander Greens 51

Mexican Pizza 52

Spice-Rubbed Salmon 54

Tuna Salad 55

Garlic and Tomatoes on Mussels 57

Spicy Cod 58

Stuffed Eggplant Shells 59

Creamy Fettuccine with Brussels Sprouts and Mushrooms 61

Sweet Onion and Sausage Spaghetti 63

Sweet Potato Steak Fries 64

White Beans with Spinach and Pan-Roasted Tomatoes 65

Arugula Salad 66

Roasted Okra 67

Raspberry Peach Pancake 68

Chocolate Truffles 69

Fresh Strawberries with Chocolate Dip 70

Cantaloupe and Mint Ice Pops 71

Grilled Pineapple Strips 73

Red Sangria 74

Lemon Pudding Cakes 75

Poached Pears 76

Apple Dumplings 77

Berry Sundae 78

Introduction

Dash Diet is the acronym for Dietary Approaches to Stop Hypertension, the major target is to reduce the sodium content of your diet by omitting table salt directly or reducing the intake through other ingredients.

Two minerals work against each other to maintain the body fluid balance; those are sodium and potassium. In perfect proportions, these two control the release and retention of fluids in the body. In the case of environmental or genetic complexities or a high sodium diet, the balance is disturbed so much that it puts our heart at risk by elevating systolic and diastolic blood pressures.

This diet comprises foods and recipes that promote lower sodium levels and higher potassium, calcium, fiber, and magnesium levels in the body. It also helps lower the overall blood pressure to an optimum level without harming the body processes. When this happens, disorders related to hypertension disappear, such as osteoporosis, diabetes, and kidney failure.

The Dash Diet works while other diets fail miserably because the body is kept full with the required nutrition. The fundamental nutrients, such as calcium, magnesium, and potassium, are elevated in the body through a wholesome diet plan, and sodium levels are also kept in control. And it is all done in a controlled, scientific, and disciplined manner without any crashes or spikes in the metabolism, ensuring a healthier you.

But anyone who wishes to get healthy and scientifically lose weight can follow it, children included.

Besides hypertension, there are several health advantages that later came to light as experts recorded the conditions people experience after choosing the diet:

- Alleviated blood pressure
- Maintained cholesterol levels
- Weight maintenance
- Reduced risks of osteoporosis
- Healthier kidneys
- Protection from cancers
- Prevention of diabetes
- Improved mental health
- Less risk of heart disease

Even if you're is not suffering from hypertension, you can adopt the Dash Diet to keep your internal systems healthy and robust.

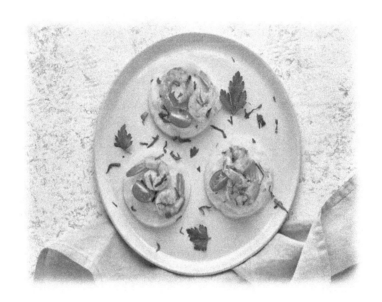

Dash Diet Recipes

GREEK YOGURT OAT PANCAKES

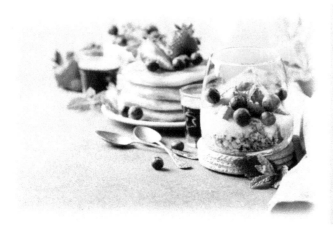

Time required:
25 minutes

Servings: 02

INGREDIENTS	STEPS FOR COOKING

6 egg whites (or ¾ cup liquid egg whites)

1 cup rolled oats

1 cup plain nonfat Greek yogurt

1 medium banana, peeled and sliced

1 teaspoon ground cinnamon

1 teaspoon baking powder

1. Blend all of the listed fixing using a blender. Warm a griddle over medium heat. Spray the skillet with nonstick cooking spray.

2. Put 1/3 cup of the mixture or batter onto the griddle. Allow to cook and flip when bubbles on the top burst, about 5 minutes. Cook again within a minute until golden brown. Repeat with the remaining batter.

3. Divide between two serving plates and enjoy.

Breakfast Bread Pudding

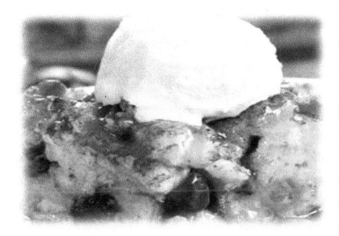

Time required:
25 minutes

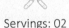

Servings: 02

INGREDIENTS

5 extra-large whole eggs

2 extra-large egg yolks

2 1/2 cups half-and-half

1/3 cup honey

1 1/2 teaspoons pure vanilla extract

2 teaspoons orange zest (2 oranges)

1/2 teaspoon kosher salt

Brioche loaf

1/2 cup golden raisins Maple syrup, to serve

STEPS FOR COOKING

1. Preheat the oven to 350 degrees F.

2. In a medium bowl, whisk together the whole eggs, egg yolks, half- and-half, honey, vanilla, orange zest, and salt. Set aside.

3. Slice the brioche loaf into 6 (1-inch) thick pieces. Lay half brioche slices flat in a 9 by 14 by 2-inch oval baking dish. Spread the raisins on top of the brioche slices, and place the remaining slices on top.

4. Make sure that the raisins are between the layers of brioche or they will burn while baking. Pour the egg mixture over the bread and allow to soak for 15 minutes, pressing down gently.

5. Bake for 55 to 60 minutes or until the pudding puffs up and the custard is set. Remove from the oven and cool slightly before serving.

Apple Pancakes

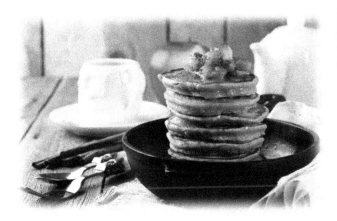

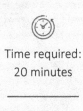

Time required:
20 minutes

Servings: 16

INGREDIENTS

¼ cup extra-virgin olive oil, divided

1 cup whole wheat flour

2 teaspoons baking powder

1 teaspoon baking soda

1 teaspoon ground cinnamon

1 cup 1% milk

2 large eggs

1 medium Gala apple, diced

2 tablespoons maple syrup

¼ cup chopped walnuts

STEPS FOR COOKING

1. Set aside 1 teaspoon of oil to use for greasing a griddle or skillet. In a large bowl, stir the flour, baking powder, baking soda, cinnamon, milk, eggs, apple, and the remaining oil.

2. Warm griddle or skillet on medium-high heat and coat with the reserved oil. Working in batches, pour in about ¼ cup of the batter for each pancake. Cook until browned on both sides.

3. Place 4 pancakes into each of 4 medium storage containers and the maple syrup in 4 small containers. Put each serving with 1 tablespoon of walnuts and drizzle with ½ tablespoon of maple syrup.

Avocado Nori Rolls

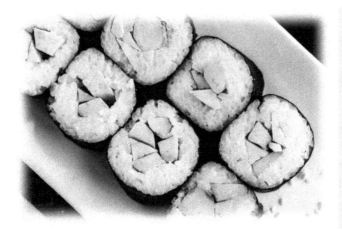

Time required:
25 minutes

Servings: 02

INGREDIENTS

2 sheets of raw or toasted sushi nori

1 large Romaine leaf cut in half down the length of the spine

2 Teaspoon of spicy miso paste

1 avocado, peeled and sliced

½ red, yellow or orange bell pepper, julienned

½ cucumber, peeled, seeded and julienned

½ cup raw sauerkraut

STEPS FOR COOKING

1. Place a sheet of nori on a sushi rolling mat or washcloth, lining it up at the end closest to you.

2. Place the Romaine leaf on the edge of the nori with the spine closest to you.

3. Spread Spicy Miso Paste on the Romaine.

4. Line the leaf with all ingredients in descending order, placing sprouts on last.

5. Roll the Nori sheet away from you, tucking the ingredients in with your fingers, and seal the roll with water or Spicy Miso Paste. Slice the roll into 6 or 8 rounds.

½ carrot, beet or zucchini, shredded

1 cup alfalfa or favorite green sprouts

1 small bowl of water for sealing roll

PERFECT GRANOLA

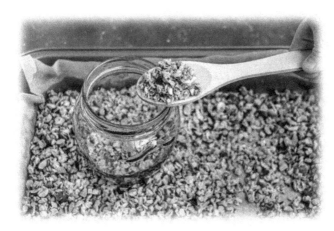

Time required:
25 minutes

Servings: 24

INGREDIENTS

¼ cup canola oil

4 tablespoons honey

1 ½ teaspoons vanilla

6 c rolled oats (old fashioned)

1 cup almonds, slivered

½ cup unsweetened coconut, shredded

2 cups bran flakes

3/4 cup walnuts, chopped

1 cup raisins

Cooking spray or parchment paper

STEPS FOR COOKING

1. Preheat the oven to 325°C.

2. In a small saucepan, put the oil, honey, and vanilla together. Cook gently over low heat, stirring regularly, or until mixed, for 5 minutes.

3. Place the remaining ingredients in a large mixing cup, except for the raisins, and combine well. Stir in the oil-honey mixture gently, ensuring the grains are uniformly covered.

4. A baking tray is lightly coated with cooking spray or filled with parchment paper. Bake in the oven until the grains are crisp and very lightly browned (about 25 mins).

5. Scatter the cereal over the baking tray. To keep the mixture from burning, stir regularly.

6. Remove from the oven the cereal and allow it to cool. Attach raisins and stir into the grain mixture uniformly.

SPINACH MUFFINS

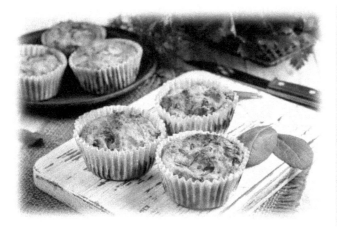

Time required:
40 minutes

Servings: 06

INGREDIENTS	STEPS FOR COOKING

INGREDIENTS

6 eggs

½ cup non-fat milk

1 cup low-fat
cheese, crumbled

4 ounces spinach

½ cup roasted red
pepper, chopped

2 ounces prosciutto,
chopped

Cooking spray

STEPS FOR COOKING

1. Mix the eggs with the milk, cheese, spinach, red pepper, and prosciutto in a bowl.

2. Grease a muffin tray with cooking spray, divide the muffin mix, introduce in the oven, and bake at 350 degrees F within 30 minutes.

3. Divide between plates and serve for breakfast.

HEALTHY BREAKFAST COOKIES

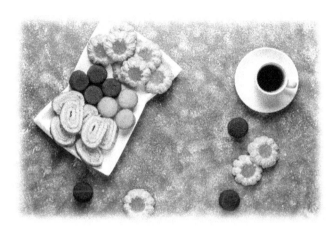

Time required:
25 minutes

Servings: 12

INGREDIENTS

1 cup creamy peanut butter (or other nut butter)

1/4 cup honey

1 teaspoon vanilla extract

2 medium ripe bananas, mashed

1/2 teaspoon salt

1 teaspoon ground cinnamon

2 1/4 cups q uick oats

1/2 cup dried cranberries or raisins

2/3 cup chopped nuts, such as

STEPS FOR COOKING

1. Preheat the oven to 325°F. Line a baking sheet with parchment paper or a Silpat.

2. In the bowl of a stand mixer fitted with the paddle attachment, beat together the peanut butter, honey, vanilla extract, mashed bananas, salt and cinnamon.

3. Add the oats, dried cranberries and nuts, then mix until combined. Scoop about 1/4-cup mounds of the cookie dough onto the baking sheet, flattening each cookie slightly. (The cookies will not spread while baking, so you can space them relatively close together.)

4. Bake the cookies for 14 to 16 minutes until they're golden brown but still soft. Remove the cookies from the

INGREDIENTS	STEPS FOR COOKING
almonds, walnuts or pistachios	oven then allow them to cool for 5 minutes on the baking sheet before transferring them to a rack to cool completely.

MEDITERRANEAN TOAST

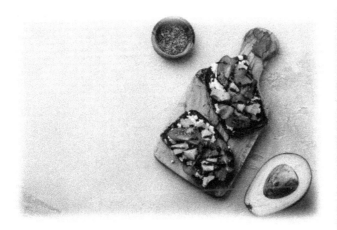

Time required:
10 minutes

Servings: 02

INGREDIENTS

1 ½ tsp. reduced-Fat crumbled feta

3 sliced Greek olives

¼ mashed avocado

1 slice good whole wheat bread

1 tbsp. roasted red pepper hummus

3 sliced cherry tomatoes

1 sliced hardboiled egg

STEPS FOR COOKING

1. First, toast the bread and top it with ¼ mashed avocado and 1 tablespoon hummus. Add the cherry tomatoes, olives, hardboiled egg, and feta.

2. To taste, season with salt and pepper.

No-Bake Breakfast Granola Bars

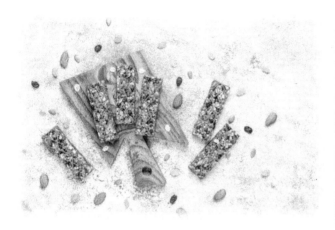

Time required:
20 minutes

Servings: 18

INGREDIENTS	STEPS FOR COOKING
2 1/2 cups toasted rice cereal 2 cups old fashioned oatmeal 1/2 cup raisins 1/2 cup firmly packed brown sugar 1/2 cup light corn syrup 1/2 cup peanut butter 1 teaspoon vanilla	1. In a large mixing cup, combine the rice cereal, oatmeal, and raisins and stir with a wooden spoon. 2. Mix the brown sugar and corn syrup together in a 1-quart saucepan. Move the heat to medium-high heat. While the mixture is brought to a boil, stirring continuously. Remove the saucepan from the fire until it is boiling. 3. In the saucepan, whisk the peanut butter and vanilla into the sugar mixture. Blend until perfectly smooth. 4. In the mixing cup, pour the peanut butter mixture over the cereal and the raisins. Mix thoroughly.

INGREDIENTS	STEPS FOR COOKING
	5. Press a 9 x 13 baking pan with the mixture. Let it totally cool and cut into 18 bars.

Strawberry Sandwich

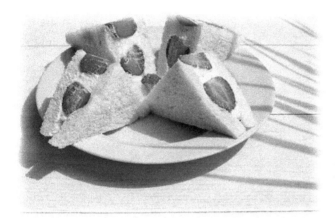

Time required:
10 minutes

Servings: 04

INGREDIENTS

8 ounces low-fat cream cheese, soft

1 tablespoon stevia

1 teaspoon lemon zest, grated

4 whole-wheat English muffins, toasted

2 cups strawberries, sliced

STEPS FOR COOKING

1. In your food processor, combine the cream cheese with the stevia and lemon zest and pulse well.

2. Spread 1 tablespoon of this mix on 1 muffin half and top with some of the sliced strawberries.

3. Repeat with the rest of the muffin halves and serve for breakfast.

4. Enjoy!

SALMON TOPPER STUFFED AVOCADOS

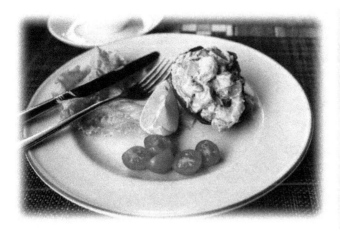

Time required:
15 minutes

Servings: 02

INGREDIENTS

*1 avocado, halved
and pitted*

*4.5 oz. True North
Salmon Toppers*

*¼ cup diced red bell
pepper*

*1 tbsp. minced
jalapeno*

*¼ cup cilantro
leaves, roughly
chopped*

1 tbsp. lime juice

Salt and pepper

STEPS FOR COOKING

1. Scoop out some of the avocado from the pitted area to widen the "bowl" area. Place the scooped avocado into a medium-size mixing bowl. Mix with a fork.

2. Add the True North Salmon Toppers, bell pepper, jalapeno, and cilantro to bowl. Pour lime juice over. Stir until everything is well mixed.

3. Scoop the Salmon Topper mixture into the avocado bowls. Season to taste with salt and pepper.

CREAMY CHICKEN BREAST

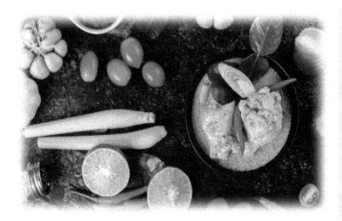

Time required:
30 minutes

Servings: 04

INGREDIENTS	STEPS FOR COOKING

1 tablespoon olive oil

A pinch of black pepper

2 pounds chicken breasts, skinless, boneless, and cubed

4 garlic cloves, minced

2 and ½ cups low-sodium chicken stock

2 cups coconut cream

½ cup low-fat parmesan, grated

1 tablespoon basil, chopped

1. Heat up a pan with the oil over medium-high heat, add chicken cubes and brown them for 3 minutes on each side.

2. Add garlic, black pepper, stock, and cream, toss, cover the pan and cook everything for 10 minutes more.

3. Add cheese and basil, toss, divide between plates and serve for lunch.

4. Enjoy!

CHICKEN, BAMBOO, AND CHESTNUTS MIX

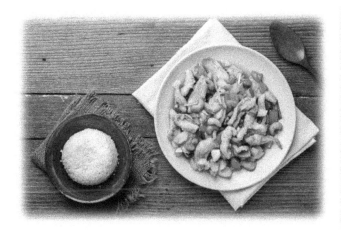

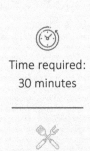

Time required:
30 minutes

Servings: 04

INGREDIENTS

1 pound chicken thighs, boneless, skinless, and cut into medium chunks

1 cup low-sodium chicken stock

1 tablespoon olive oil

2 tablespoons coconut aminos

1-inch ginger, grated

1 carrot, sliced

2 garlic cloves, minced

8 ounces canned bamboo shoots, drained

STEPS FOR COOKING

1. Heat up a pan with the oil over medium-high heat, add chicken, stir, and brown for 4 minutes on each side.

2. Add the stock, aminos, ginger, carrot, garlic, bamboo, and chestnuts, toss, cover the pan, then cook everything over medium heat for 12 minutes.

3. Divide everything between plates and serve.

4. Enjoy!

INGREDIENTS	STEPS FOR COOKING
8 ounces water chestnuts	

SUNSHINE WRAP

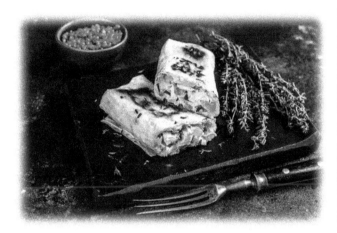

Time required:
25 minutes

Servings: 04

INGREDIENTS

8 oz chicken breast

½ cup celery, diced

2/3 cup canned mandarin oranges, drained

¼ cup onion, minced

2 tablespoons mayonnaise

1 teaspoon soy sauce

¼ teaspoon garlic powder

¼ teaspoon black pepper

1 large whole wheat tortilla

STEPS FOR COOKING

1. Cook chicken breast in a non-stick pan on medium-high heat until done all through (165oF internal temperature). Cut into 1/2-inch cubes until the chicken has cooled enough to treat.

2. Combine the chicken, celery, oranges, and onions in a medium dish. Add the mayonnaise, soy sauce, pepper, and garlic. Mix softly until evenly covered with the chicken mixture.

3. On a clean cutting board or wide pan, position the tortilla. Break the tortilla into four quarters with a knife or tidy kitchen scissors. On each tortilla fifth, position 1-lettuce leaf, trimming the leaf to hang over the tortilla.

4. In the center of each lettuce leaf, place 1/4 of the chicken mixture. Roll

4 large lettuce leaves, washed and dried

tortillas up into a cone, forming the cone's opening with the two straight sides going together with the curved end. Eat the wrap like a sandwich.

5. Leftovers should be refrigerated within 2 hours.

PESTO AND MOZZARELLA STUFFED PORTOBELLO MUSHROOM CAPS

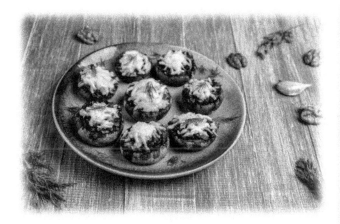

Time required:
20 minutes

Servings: 04

INGREDIENTS

2 portobello mushroom caps

1 small Roma tomato, diced

2 tablespoons pesto

¼ cup shredded low-fat mozzarella cheese

STEPS FOR COOKING

1. Use a damp cloth to clean mushrooms, then remove stems by twisting gently.

2. Divide pesto evenly between 2 mushroom caps.

3. Top with diced tomato and shredded cheese.

4. Set the oven to 400 F and bake for 15 minutes.

CREAMY PUMPKIN PASTA

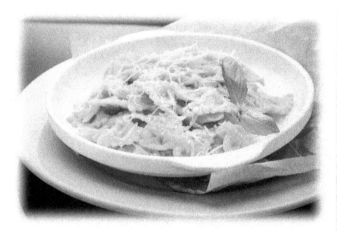

Time required:
45 minutes

Servings: 06

INGREDIENTS

1-pound whole-grain linguine

1 tablespoon olive oil

3 garlic cloves, peeled and minced

2 tablespoons chopped fresh sage

1½ cups pumpkin purée

1 cup unsalted vegetable stock

½ cup low-fat evaporated milk

¾ teaspoon kosher or sea salt

½ teaspoon ground black pepper

STEPS FOR COOKING

1. Cook the whole-grain linguine in a large pot of boiled water.

2. Reserve ½ cup of pasta water and drain the rest, then set the pasta aside.

3. Warm-up olive oil over medium heat in a large skillet. Add the garlic and sage and sauté for 1 to 2 minutes, until soft and fragrant. Whisk in the pumpkin purée, stock, milk, and reserved pasta water and simmer for 4 to 5 minutes, until thickened.

4. Whisk in the salt, black pepper, nutmeg, and cayenne pepper and half of the Parmesan cheese. Stir in the cooked whole-grain linguine.

½ teaspoon ground nutmeg

¼ teaspoon ground cayenne pepper

½ cup freshly grated Parmesan cheese, divided

5. Evenly divide the pasta among 6 bowls and top with the remaining Parmesan cheese.

Avocado Cup with Egg

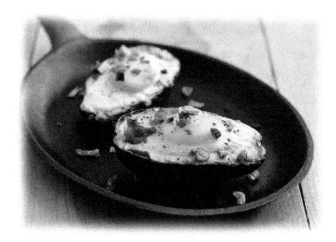

Time required:
5 minutes

___

Servings: 04

INGREDIENTS

4 tsp. parmesan cheese

1 chopped stalk scallion

4 dashes pepper

4 dashes paprika

2 ripe avocados

4 medium eggs

STEPS FOR COOKING

1. Preheat oven to 375 0F. Slice avocadoes in half and discard the seed.

2. Slice the rounded portions of the avocado to make it level, then sit well on a baking sheet.

3. Place avocadoes on a baking sheet and crack one egg in each hole of the avocado. Season each egg evenly with pepper and paprika. Bake within 25 minutes or until eggs are cooked to your liking. Serve with a sprinkle of parmesan.

Chicken Vegetable Soup

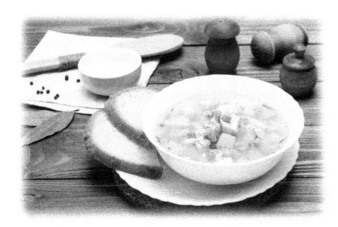

Time required:
55 minutes

Servings: 04

INGREDIENTS

1 tablespoon butter

1/2 cup onion finely diced

2 carrots peeled, halved lengthwise and sliced

2 stalks celery thinly sliced

2 teaspoons minced garlic

3 cups cooked chicken shredded or cubed salt and pepper to taste

15 ounce can diced tomatoes do not drain

STEPS FOR COOKING

1. Melt the butter in a large pot over medium high heat. Add the onion, carrots and celery to the pot.

2. Cook for 5-6 minutes or until softened. Add the garlic and cook for 30 seconds more. Season with salt and pepper to taste.

3. Add the chicken, tomatoes, tomato sauce, Italian seasoning, chicken broth and potato to the pot; bring to a simmer.

4. Cook for 20-25 minutes or until potatoes are tender. Taste and add salt and pepper as desired.

5. Stir in the corn and green beans and cook for 5 minutes more.

6. Sprinkle with parsley and serve.

INGREDIENTS

8 ounce can tomato sauce

1 teaspoon Italian seasoning

6 cups chicken broth

1 large Russet potato peeled and cut into 1/2 inch cubes

1/2 cup frozen corn

1/2 cup diced green beans fresh or frozen

2 tablespoons chopped fresh parsley

STEPS FOR COOKING

Salsa Chicken

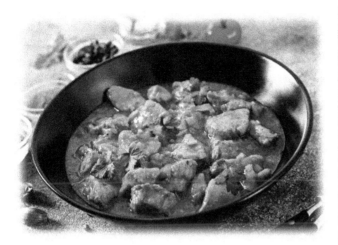

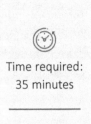

Time required:
35 minutes

Servings: 04

INGREDIENTS

1 cup mild salsa, no-salt-added

½ teaspoon cumin, ground

Black pepper

1 tablespoon chipotle paste

1-pound chicken thighs, skinless and boneless

2 cups corn

Juice of 1 lime

½ tablespoon olive oil

2 tablespoons cilantro, chopped

STEPS FOR COOKING

1. In a pot, combine the salsa with cumin, black pepper, chipotle paste, chicken thighs, and corn, toss, bring to a simmer and cook over medium heat for 25 minutes.

2. Add lime juice, oil, cherry tomatoes, and avocado, toss, divide into bowls and serve for lunch.

3. Enjoy!

INGREDIENTS

*1 cup cherry
tomatoes, halved*

*1 small avocado,
pitted, peeled, and
cubed*

Sweet Potato Soup

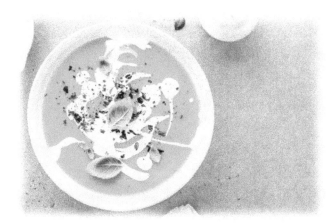

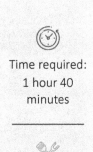

Time required:
1 hour 40
minutes

Servings: 06

INGREDIENTS	STEPS FOR COOKING

4 big sweet potatoes

28 ounces veggie stock

A pinch of black pepper

¼ teaspoon nutmeg, ground

1/3 cup low-sodium heavy cream

1. Put the sweet potatoes on a lined baking sheet, bake them at 350 degrees F for 1 hour and 30 minutes, cool them down, peel, roughly chop them, and put them in a pot.

2. Add stock, nutmeg, cream, and pepper pulse well using an immersion blender, heat the soup over medium heat, cook for 10 minutes, ladle into bowls and serve.

3. Enjoy!

PEAR, TURKEY AND CHEESE SANDWICH

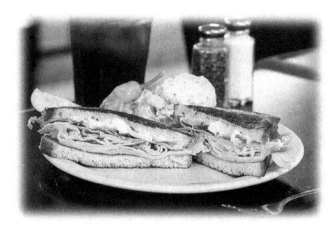

Time required:
10 minutes

Servings: 06

INGREDIENTS	STEPS FOR COOKING
2 slices multi-grain or rye sandwich bread *2 tsp Dijon-style mustard* *2 slices (1 oz. each) reduced-sodium cooked or smoked turkey* *1 USA pear, cored and thinly sliced* *1/4 cup shredded low-fat mozzarella cheese* *Coarsely ground pepper*	1. Spread 1-teaspoon of mustard on each slice of bread. Place each slice of bread with one slice of turkey. Arrange the turkey pear slices and sprinkle each with 2-tablespoons of cheese. Sprinkle spice over it. 2. Broil, 2 to 3 minutes or until turkey and pears are hot and cheese melts, 4 to 6 inches from the sun. 3. Halve each sandwich and serve the open face in half.

Turkey Meatloaf

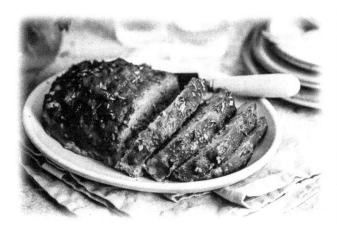

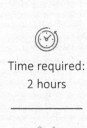

Time required:
2 hours

Servings: 02

INGREDIENTS

1 slice 100% whole wheat bread, crust removed and torn into small pieces

1/4 cup low-sodium chicken stock

1 1/4 pounds lean ground turkey

1 large egg

1/4 cup finely chopped onion

1/4 cup finely chopped bell pepper

1/4 cup chopped fresh parsley

1 teaspoon horseradish

STEPS FOR COOKING

1. Preheat the oven to 350°F. Place all the ingredients in a big bowl and combine until the ingredients are properly incorporated together with your fingertips, being vigilant not to overmix.

2. Grease a 9-by 5-inch loaf pan (or deep baking dish) lightly with a spray of olive oil. In a loaf, shape the meat mixture and put it in the pan. Bake uncovered for an hour or two.

3. Remove from the oven until the meatloaf is baked and let cool for about 10 minutes. To detach it from the plate, run a butter knife around the sides, invert it into a large serving bowl, and slice it to eat.

INGREDIENTS

1 teaspoon Dijon mustard

1 teaspoon Worcestershire sauce

1/2 teaspoon sea salt

1/4 teaspoon black pepper

STEPS FOR COOKING

Pesto Shrimp Pasta

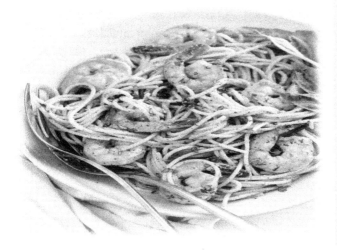

Time required:
27 minutes

Servings: 04

INGREDIENTS

1/8 teaspoon freshly cracked pepper

1 cup dried orzo

4 tsp packaged pesto sauce mix

1 lemon, halved

1/8 teaspoon coarse salt

1-pound medium shrimp, thawed

1 medium zucchini, halved lengthwise and sliced

2 tablespoons olive oil, divided

1-ounce shaved Parmesan cheese

STEPS FOR COOKING

1. Prepare orzo pasta concerning package directions, then drain; reserving ¼ cup of the pasta cooking water. Mix 1 teaspoon of the pesto mix into the kept cooking water and set aside.

2. Mix 3 teaspoons of the pesto mix plus 1 tablespoon of olive oil in a large plastic bag. Seal and shake to mix. Put the shrimp in the bag; seal and turn to coat. Set aside.

3. Sauté zucchini in a big skillet over moderate heat for 1 to 2 minutes, stirring repeatedly. Put the pesto-marinated shrimp in the skillet and cook for 5 minutes or until shrimp is dense.

4. Put the cooked pasta in the skillet with the zucchini and shrimp combination. Stir in the kept pasta water until absorbed, grating up any seasoning in the bottom of the pan. Season with pepper and salt. Squeeze the lemon over the pasta. Top with Parmesan, then serve.

Hot Chicken Wings

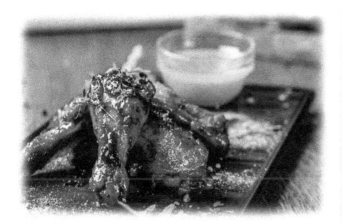

Time required:
40 minutes

_____

Servings: 04

INGREDIENTS	STEPS FOR COOKING

10 - 20 chicken wings
½ stick margarine
1 bottle Durkee hot sauce
2 Tablespoons honey
10 shakes Tabasco sauce
2 Tablespoons cayenne pepper

1. Warm canola oil in a deep pot. Deep-fry the wings until cooked, approximately 20 minutes. Mix the hot sauce, honey, Tabasco, and cayenne pepper in a medium bowl. Mix well.

2. Place the cooked wings on paper towels. Drain the excess oil. Mix the chicken wings in the sauce until coated evenly.

Spinach-Orzo Salad with Chickpeas

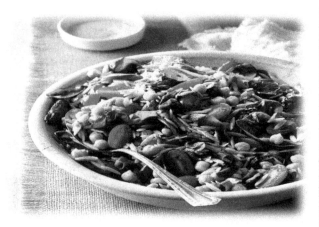

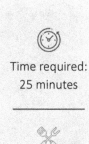

Time required:
25 minutes

Servings: 12

INGREDIENTS	STEPS FOR COOKING

1 can (14-1/2 ounces) reduced-sodium chicken broth

1-1/2 cups uncooked whole wheat orzo pasta

4 cups fresh baby spinach

2 cups grape tomatoes, halved

2 cans (15 ounces each) chickpeas or garbanzo beans, rinsed and drained

3/4 cup chopped fresh parsley

1. In a large saucepan, bring broth to a boil. Stir in orzo; return to a boil. Reduce heat; simmer, covered, until al dente, 8-10 minutes.

2. In a large bowl, toss spinach and warm orzo, allowing spinach to wilt slightly. Add tomatoes, chickpeas, parsley and green onions.

3. Whisk together dressing ingredients. Toss with salad.

2 green onions, chopped

Dressing:

1/4 cup olive oil

3 tablespoons lemon juice

3/4 teaspoon salt

1/4 teaspoon garlic powder

1/4 teaspoon hot pepper sauce

1/4 teaspoon pepper

BLACK BEAN AND SWEET POTATO RICE BOWLS

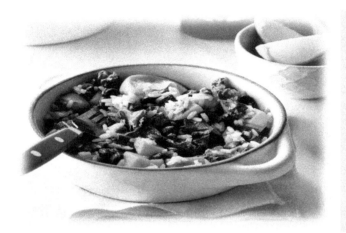

Time required:
30 minutes

_____

Servings: 04

INGREDIENTS	STEPS FOR COOKING

INGREDIENTS

3/4 cup uncooked long grain rice

1/4 teaspoon garlic salt

1-1/2 cups water

3 tablespoons olive oil, divided

1 large sweet potato, peeled and diced

1 medium red onion, finely chopped

4 cups chopped fresh kale (tough stems removed)

1 can (15 ounces) black beans, rinsed and drained

STEPS FOR COOKING

1. Place rice, garlic salt and water in a large saucepan; bring to a boil. Reduce heat; simmer, covered, until water is absorbed and rice is tender, 15-20 minutes. Remove from heat; let stand 5 minutes.

2. Meanwhile, in a large skillet, heat 2 tablespoons oil over medium- high heat; saute sweet potato 8 minutes. Add onion; cook and stir until potato is tender, 4-6 minutes. Add kale; cook and stir until tender, 3-5 minutes. Stir in beans; heat through.

3. Gently stir 2 tablespoons chili sauce and remaining oil into rice; add to potato mixture. If desired, serve with lime wedges and additional chili sauce.

2 tablespoons sweet
chili sauce

Lime wedges,
optional

Additional sweet
chili sauce, optional

Paprika Lamb Chops

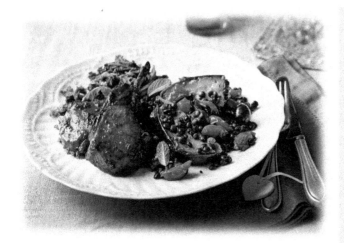

Time required:
25 minutes

Servings: 04

INGREDIENTS	STEPS FOR COOKING

INGREDIENTS

1 lamb rack, cut into chops

pepper to taste

1 tablespoon paprika

1/2 cup cumin powder

1/2 teaspoon chili powder

STEPS FOR COOKING

1. Add paprika, cumin, chili, pepper into a bowl, then stir.
2. Add lamb chops and rub the mixture.
3. Heat grill over medium-temperature and add lamb chops, cook for 5 minutes.
4. Flip and cook for 5 minutes more, flip again.
5. Cook for 2 minutes, flip and cook for 2 minutes more.
6. Serve and enjoy!

Zucchini Beef Sauté with Coriander Greens

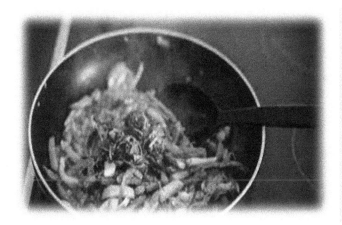

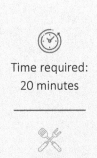

Time required:
20 minutes

Servings: 04

INGREDIENTS

1 zucchini, cut into
2-inch strips

¼ cup parsley,
chopped

3 garlic cloves,
minced

2 tablespoons
tamari sauce

4 tablespoons
avocado oil

STEPS FOR COOKING

1. Add 2 tablespoons avocado oil in a frying pan over high heat.

2. Place strips of beef and brown for a few minutes on high heat.

3. Once the meat is brown, add zucchini strips and sauté until tender.

4. Once tender, add tamari sauce, garlic, parsley and let them sit for a few minutes more.

5. Serve immediately and enjoy!

Mexican Pizza

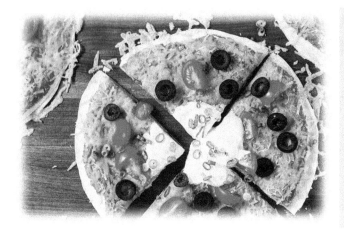

Time required:
20 minutes

Servings: 06

INGREDIENTS	STEPS FOR COOKING

INGREDIENTS

1/2 cup rinsed and drained canned black beans

1 tablespoon canned chipotle pepper sauce

3 tablespoons water

1 (12-inch) prebaked 100% whole wheat thin-crust pizza

1 small zucchini, thinly sliced in rounds

1/2 cup thinly sliced red onion

1/2 cup sliced red bell pepper

STEPS FOR COOKING

1. Preheat the oven to 400 F. In a food processor or blender, combine the chipotle salsa, black beans, and water. Puree until it hits Only smooth. Spread the mixture uniformly over the pie crust.

2. Cover with rounds of zucchini, then onions and bell peppers, and eventually cheese. Sprinkle on top of oregano and cook for about 15 minutes, or until the cheese is browned and bubbled.

1/2 cup shredded
skim mozzarella
cheese
1/2 teaspoon dried
oregano

Spice-Rubbed Salmon

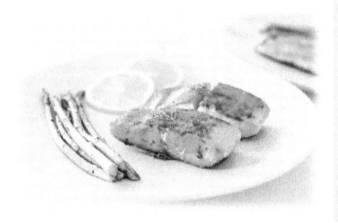

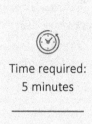
Time required:
5 minutes

Servings: 04

INGREDIENTS	STEPS FOR COOKING

INGREDIENTS

2 teaspoons chili powder

1 teaspoon ground cumin

1 teaspoon brown sugar

1/8 teaspoon sea salt

1/8 teaspoon cracked black pepper

4 (4-ounce) salmon fillets

Juice of 1/2 orange

2 tablespoons extra virgin olive oil

STEPS FOR COOKING

1. Blend the chili powder, cumin, sugar, salt, and pepper in a shallow cup. Rub the mixture by hand onto each salmon fillet.

2. Over medium pressure, heat the oil in a nonstick pan. When the oil is heated, add two fillets to the pan at a time, skin side down, and cook for 1 to 2 minutes. Then turn the fillets over and squeeze them with the orange juice.

3. Cook until the fillets are flaky for another 1 to 2 minutes and can be separated with a fork. With the second set of fillets, repeat the operation. Immediately serve.

Tuna Salad

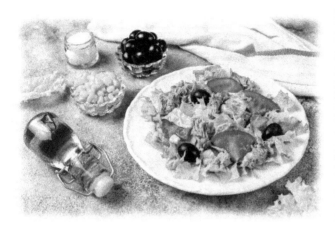

Time required:
20 minutes

Servings: 08

INGREDIENTS	STEPS FOR COOKING

1/4 cup chopped celery

1/2 jalapeño chile pepper, seeded and chopped

1/4 cup chopped Roma tomato

1/4 cup chopped red onion

2 cans albacore tuna in water, no salt added, drained

1 teaspoon brown mustard

3 tablespoons low-fat plain Greek yogurt

1. Combine the celery, chili, tomato, and onion in a medium dish.
2. Combine the salmon, vinegar, yogurt, and pepper together until well blended. Cover with avocado slices in the salad, and eat.

1/8 teaspoon cracked black pepper

1 small avocado, thinly sliced

GARLIC AND TOMATOES ON MUSSELS

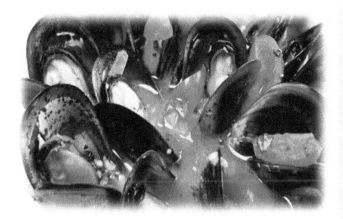

Time required:
30 minutes

Servings: 06

INGREDIENTS

¼ cup white wine

½ cup of water

3 Roma tomatoes, chopped

2 cloves of garlic, minced

1 bay leaf

2 pounds mussels, scrubbed

½ cup fresh parsley, chopped

1 tbsp oil

Pepper

STEPS FOR COOKING

1. Warm a pot on medium-high fire within 3 minutes. Put oil and stir around to coat the pot with oil. Sauté the garlic, bay leaf, and tomatoes for 5 minutes.

2. Add remaining ingredients except for parsley and mussels. Mix well. Add mussels. Cover, and boil for 5 minutes.

3. Serve with a sprinkle of parsley and discard any unopened mussels.

Spicy Cod

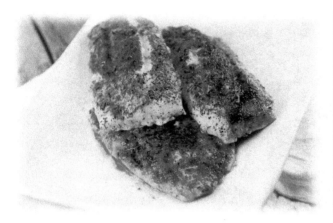

Time required:
45 minutes

Servings: 04

INGREDIENTS	STEPS FOR COOKING

2 pounds cod fillets

1 Tablespoon flavorless oil (olive, canola, or sunflower)

2 cups low sodium salsa

2 tablespoons fresh chopped parsley

1. Warm oven to 350 F. In a large, deep baking dish, drizzle the oil along the bottom. Place the cod fillets in the dish. Pour the salsa over the fish.

2. Cover with foil for 20 minutes. Remove the foil last 10 minutes of cooking. Bake in the oven for 20 – 30 minutes, until the fish is flaky. Serve with white or brown rice.

3. Garnish with parsley.

Stuffed Eggplant Shells

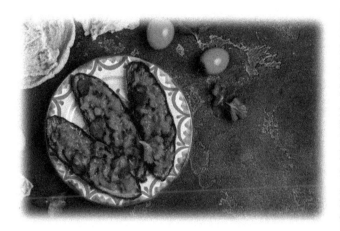

Time required:
35 minutes

Servings: 02

INGREDIENTS

1 medium eggplant

1 cup of water

1 tablespoon olive oil

4 oz. cooked white beans

1/4 cup onion, chopped

1/2 cup red, green, or yellow bell peppers, chopped

1 cup canned unsalted tomatoes

1/4 cup tomatoes liquid

1/4 cup celery, chopped

STEPS FOR COOKING

1. Prepare the oven to 350 degrees F to preheat. Grease a baking dish with cooking spray and set it aside. Trim and cut the eggplant into half, lengthwise. Scoop out the pulp using a spoon and leave the shell about ¼ inch thick.

2. Place the shells in the baking dish with their cut side up. Add water to the bottom of the dish. Dice the eggplant pulp into cubes and set them aside. Add oil to an iron skillet and heat it over medium heat. Stir in onions, peppers, chopped eggplant, tomatoes, celery, mushrooms, and tomato juice.

3. Cook for 10 minutes on simmering heat, then stirs in beans, black pepper, and breadcrumbs. Divide this mixture into the eggplant

1 cup fresh mushrooms, sliced

3/4 cup whole-wheat breadcrumbs

Freshly ground black pepper, to taste

CREAMY FETTUCCINE WITH BRUSSELS SPROUTS AND MUSHROOMS

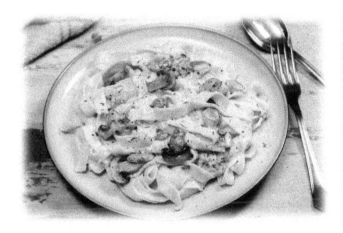

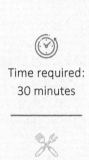

Time required:
30 minutes

Servings: 06

INGREDIENTS

12 ounces whole-wheat fettuccine

1 tablespoon extra-virgin olive oil

4 cups sliced mixed mushrooms, such as cremini, oyster and/or shiitake

4 cups thinly sliced Brussels sprouts

1 tablespoon minced garlic

½ cup dry sherry (see Note), or 2 tablespoons sherry vinegar

2 cups low-fat milk

STEPS FOR COOKING

1. Cook pasta in a large pot of boiling water until tender, 8 to 10 minutes. Drain, return to the pot and set aside. Meanwhile, heat oil in a large skillet over medium heat. Add mushrooms and Brussels sprouts and cook, stirring often, until the mushrooms release their li q uid, 8 to 10 minutes. Add garlic and cook, stirring, until fragrant, about 1 minute.

2. Add sherry (or vinegar), scraping up any brown bits; bring to a boil and cook, stirring, until almost evaporated, 10 seconds (if using vinegar) or about 1 minute (if using sherry).

2 tablespoons all-purpose flour

½ teaspoon salt

½ teaspoon freshly ground pepper

1 cup finely shredded Asiago cheese, plus more for garnish

3. Whisk milk and flour in a bowl; add to the skillet with salt and pepper. Cook, stirring, until the sauce bubbles and thickens, about 2 minutes.

4. Stir in Asiago until melted. Add the sauce to the pasta; gently toss.

5. Serve with more cheese, if desired.

Sweet Onion and Sausage Spaghetti

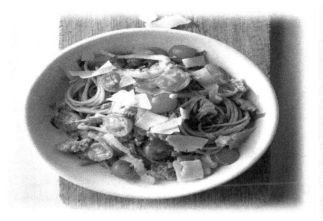

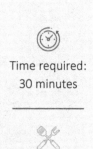

Time required:
30 minutes

Servings: 04

INGREDIENTS	STEPS FOR COOKING

INGREDIENTS

6 ounces uncooked whole wheat spaghetti

3/4 pound Italian turkey sausage links, casings removed

2 teaspoons olive oil

1 sweet onion, thinly sliced

1 pint cherry tomatoes, halved

1/2 cup loosely packed fresh basil leaves, thinly sliced

1/2 cup half-and-half cream

Shaved Parmesan cheese, optional

STEPS FOR COOKING

1. Cook spaghetti according to package directions. Meanwhile, in a large nonstick skillet over medium heat, cook sausage in oil for 5 minutes. Add onion; cook 8-10 minutes longer or until meat is no longer pink and onion is tender.

2. Stir in tomatoes and basil; heat through. Add cream; bring to a boil. Drain spaghetti; toss with sausage mixture.

3. Garnish with cheese if desired.

SWEET POTATO STEAK FRIES

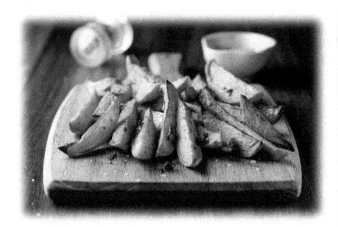

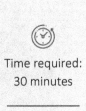

Time required:
30 minutes

Servings: 04

INGREDIENTS

Olive oil in a pump sprayer

3 large orange-fleshed sweet potatoes (1½ pounds)

½ teaspoon kosher salt

¼ teaspoon freshly ground black pepper

STEPS FOR COOKING

1. Preheat the oven to 425 F. Using oil to spray a large rimmed baking sheet.

2. Peel the sweet potatoes and cut each one into 6 long wedges lengthwise. Spread out on the baking sheet in a single layer, then oil spray, toss and spray again. For 15 minutes, bake.

3. Switch the fries and bake for about 15 more minutes, until lightly browned and soft. Use salt and pepper to season, toss well, and serve sweet.

WHITE BEANS WITH SPINACH AND PAN-ROASTED TOMATOES

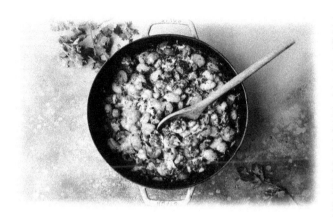

Time required:
25 minutes

Servings: 02

INGREDIENTS

1 tablespoon olive oil

4 small plum tomatoes, halved lengthwise

10 ounces frozen spinach, defrosted and squeezed of excess water

2 garlic cloves, thinly sliced

2 tablespoons water

¼ teaspoon freshly ground black pepper

1 can white beans, drained

Juice of 1 lemon

STEPS FOR COOKING

1. Heat up the oil in a skillet over medium-high. Put the tomatoes, cut-side down, and cook within 3 to 5 minutes; turn and cook within 1 minute more. Transfer to a plate.

2. Reduce heat to medium and add the spinach, garlic, water, and pepper to the skillet. Cook, tossing until the spinach is heated through, 2 to 3 minutes.

3. Return the tomatoes to the skillet, put the white beans and lemon juice, and toss until heated through 1 to 2 minutes.

ARUGULA SALAD

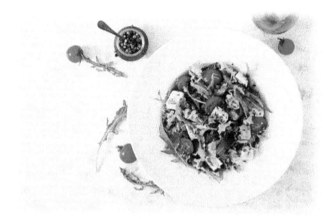

Time required:
5 minutes

Servings: 04

INGREDIENTS

¼ cup pomegranate seeds

5 cups baby arugula

6 tablespoons green onions, chopped

1 tablespoon balsamic vinegar

2 tablespoons olive oil

3 tablespoons pine nuts

½ shallot, chopped

STEPS FOR COOKING

1. In a salad bowl, combine the arugula with the pomegranate and the other ingredients.

2. Toss and serve.

ROASTED OKRA

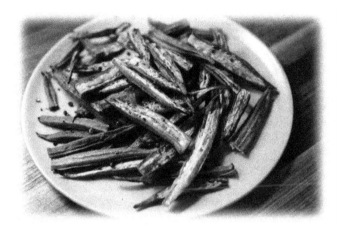

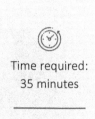

Time required:
35 minutes

Servings: 04

INGREDIENTS	STEPS FOR COOKING

1 pound Okra, fresh

2 tablespoons Extra virgin olive oil

.125 teaspoon Cayenne pepper, ground

1 teaspoon Paprika

.25 teaspoon Garlic powder

1. Warm the oven to Fahrenheit 450 degrees and prepare a large baking sheet. Cut the okra into pieces appropriate 1/2-inch in size.

2. Place the okra on the baking pan and top it with the olive oil and seasonings, giving it a good toss until evenly coated. Roast the okra in the heated oven until it is tender and lightly browned and seared.

3. Serve immediately while hot.

RASPBERRY PEACH PANCAKE

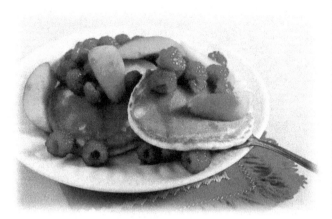

Time required:
45 minutes

Servings: 04

INGREDIENTS

½ teaspoon sugar

½ cup raspberries

½ cup fat-free milk

½ cup all-purpose flour

¼ cup vanilla yogurt

1/8 teaspoon iodized salt

1 tablespoon butter

2 medium peeled, thinly sliced peaches

3 lightly beaten organic eggs

STEPS FOR COOKING

1. Preheat oven to 400 °F. Toss peaches and raspberries with sugar in a bowl. Melt butter on a 9-inch round baking plate. Mix eggs, milk, plus salt in a small bowl until blended; whisk in the flour.

2. Remove the round baking plate from the oven, tilt to coat the bottom and sides with the melted butter; pour in the flour mixture.

3. Put it in the oven until it becomes brownish and puffed. Remove the pancake from the oven. Serve immediately with more raspberries and vanilla yogurt.

Chocolate Truffles

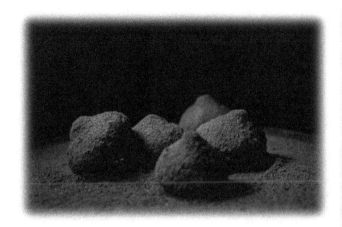

Time required:
25 minutes

Servings: 02

INGREDIENTS

For the Truffles:

½ cup cacao powder

¼ cup chia seeds

¼ cup flaxseed meal

¼ cup maple syrup

1 cup flour

2 tablespoons almond milk

For the Coatings:

Cacao powder Chia seeds Flour

Shredded coconut, unsweetened

STEPS FOR COOKING

1. Place all the fixing for the truffle in a blender; pulse until it is thoroughly blended; transfer contents to a bowl. Form into chocolate balls, then cover with the coating ingredients.

2. Serve immediately.

FRESH STRAWBERRIES WITH CHOCOLATE DIP

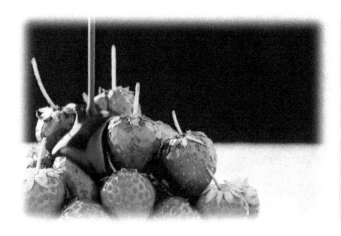

Time required:
30 minutes

Servings: 04

INGREDIENTS	STEPS FOR COOKING
½ cup low-fat (2%) canned evaporated milk	1. In a tiny saucepan, carry the evaporated milk to a boil over medium heat. Remove from the heat, then add the chocolate. Let it stand for about 3 minutes before the chocolate softens. Until smooth, whisk.
5 ounces bittersweet chocolate (about 60% cacao content), finely chopped	2. Divide the mixture of chocolate into four tiny ramekins. To dip, serve the strawberries with the chocolate mixture.
24 strawberries, unhulled	

Cantaloupe and Mint Ice Pops

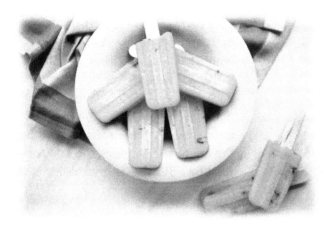

Time required:
30 minutes

Servings: 04

INGREDIENTS	STEPS FOR COOKING

3 cups peeled, seeded, and cubed ripe cantaloupe

½ cup amber agave nectar

2 tablespoons fresh lemon juice

1 tablespoon finely chopped fresh mint

1. Have eight ice pop molds ready. In a food processor or blender, purée 2 1/2 cups of the cantaloupe cubes. Transfer to a bowl. Pulse in the food processor or blender (or slice by hand) the remaining 1/2 cup of cantaloupe cubes until finely chopped, and add to the puree. Apply the agave, lemon juice, and mint to the whisk.

2. Divide the puree between the ice pop molds and cover the lid of each mold. Freeze for at least 4 hours, until the pops are strong. (The pops can be kept in the freezer for up to 1 week.)

3. Rinse the pop mold under lukewarm water to serve, then remove the pop from the mold. Frozen serve.

4. Cantaloupe and Mint Granita: In the freezer, put a metal baking dish or

INGREDIENTS	STEPS FOR COOKING

cake pan and a metal fork until very cold, approximately 15 minutes. The whole cantaloupe purée. To combine well, add the agave and the lemon juice and pulse. Only to mix, add the mint and pulse. Pour into the metal dish and freeze for around 1 hour until the mixture is icy along the sides of the bowl. Stir the ice crystals into the middle using the cold fork.

5. Freeze again, around 1 hour more, until icy, and stir again; the mixture becomes more solid. Freeze for about 1 hour more, until the consistency is slushy. Freeze for up to 4 hours before serving. Using the fork's tines to scrape the mixture into frozen slush just before serving. Serve in chilled bowls immediately.

GRILLED PINEAPPLE STRIPS

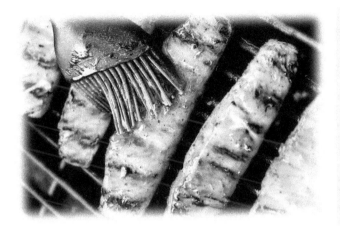

Time required:
20 minutes

Servings: 06

INGREDIENTS

Vegetable oil

Dash of iodized salt

1 pineapple

1 tablespoon lime juice extract

1 tablespoon olive oil

1 tablespoon raw honey

3 tablespoons brown sugar

STEPS FOR COOKING

1. Peel the pineapple, remove the eyes of the fruit, and discard the core. Slice lengthwise, forming six wedges. Mix the rest of the fixing in a bowl until blended.

2. Brush the coating mixture on the pineapple (reserve some for basting). Grease an oven or outdoor grill rack with vegetable oil.

3. Place the pineapple wedges on the grill rack and heat for a few minutes per side until golden brownish, basting it frequently with a reserved glaze. Serve on a platter.

Red Sangria

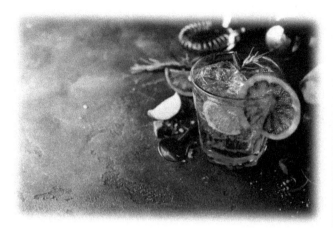

Time required:
5 minutes

Servings: 08

INGREDIENTS

1 (750 mL) bottle
Spanish red table
wine

1/4 cup brandy

1/4 cup Cointreau

1/2 cup orange juice

1 cup pomegranate
juice

2 oranges, thinly
sliced

2 Granny Smith
apples, thinly sliced

1 1/2 cups seltzer,
mineral water

STEPS FOR COOKING

1. Stir together the champagne, brandy, Cointreau, and fruit juices in a big pitcher.

2. Add the sliced fruit and chill for at least 30 minutes in the refrigerator before eating. Just prior to serving, add the seltzer, sparkling water, or club soda.

Lemon Pudding Cakes

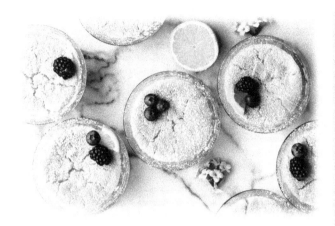

Time required:
50 minutes

Servings: 04

INGREDIENTS	STEPS FOR COOKING

INGREDIENTS

2 eggs

1/4 teaspoon salt

3/4 cup sugar

1 cup skim milk

1/3 cup freshly squeezed lemon juice

3 tablespoons all-purpose flour

1 tablespoon finely grated lemon peel

1 tablespoon melted butter

STEPS FOR COOKING

1. Warm oven at 350 degrees F. Grease the custard cups with cooking oil. Whisk egg whites with salt and ¼ cup sugar in a mixer until it forms stiff peaks. Beat egg yolks with ½ cup sugar until mixed.

2. Stir in lemon juice, milk, butter, flour, and lemon peel. Mix it until smooth. Fold in the egg white mixture. Divide the batter into the custard cups. Bake them for 40 minutes until golden from the top.

3. Serve.

POACHED PEARS

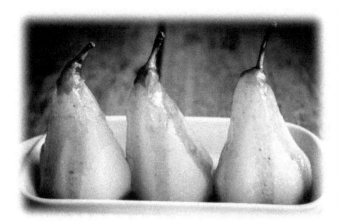

Time required:
45 minutes

Servings: 04

INGREDIENTS	STEPS FOR COOKING

INGREDIENTS

¼ cup apple juice extract

½ cup fresh raspberries

1 cup of orange juice extract

1 teaspoon cinnamon, ground

1 teaspoon ground nutmeg

2 tablespoons orange zest

4 whole pears, peeled, destemmed, core removed

STEPS FOR COOKING

1. In a bowl, combine the fruit juices, nutmeg, and cinnamon, and then stir evenly. In a shallow pan, pour the fruit juice mixture, and set it to medium fire.

2. Adjust the heat to simmer within 30 minutes; turn pears frequently to maintain poaching, do not boil. Transfer poached pears to a serving bowl; garnish with orange zest and raspberries.

APPLE DUMPLINGS

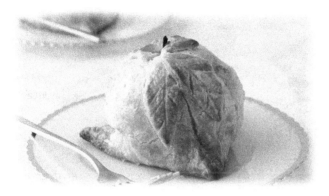

Time required:
40 minutes

Servings: 06

INGREDIENTS

Dough:

1 tablespoon butter

1 teaspoon honey

1 cup whole-wheat flour

2 tablespoons buckwheat flour

2 tablespoons rolled oats

2 tablespoons brandy or apple liquor

Apple Filling:

6 large tart apples, thinly sliced

1 teaspoon nutmeg

2 tablespoons honey

Zest of one lemon

STEPS FOR COOKING

1. Warm oven to heat at 350 degrees F. Combine flours with oats, honey, and butter in a food processor. Pulse this mixture for few times, then stirs in apple liquor or brandy. Mix until it forms a ball. Wrap it in a plastic sheet.

2. Refrigerate for 2 hours. Mix apples with honey, nutmeg, and lemon zest, then set it aside. Spread the dough into ¼ inch thick sheet. Cut it into 8-inch circles and layer the greased muffin cups with the dough circles.

3. Divide the apple mixture into the muffin cups and seal the dough from the top. Bake for 30 minutes at 350 degrees F until golden brown. Enjoy.

BERRY SUNDAE

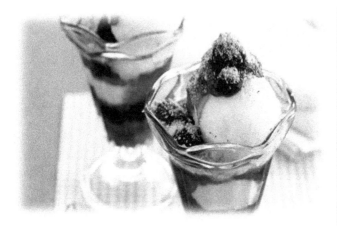

Time required:
15 minutes

Servings: 06

INGREDIENTS

1 1/2 cups coarsely
chopped
strawberries
1 1/2 cups
blueberries
1 1/2 cups
raspberries
1 1/2 tablespoons
balsamic vinegar
Pinch of cracked
black pepper
1 1/2 teaspoons
grated lemon zest1
1/2 teaspoons
grated orange zest
Juice of 1/2 orange
1/2 teaspoon vanilla
extract

STEPS FOR COOKING

1. In a big pot over medium heat, put all
    the ingredients except the yogurt and
    almonds and cook until the liquid
    starts to bubble.

2. Reduce the heat to low and simmer
    for about 15 minutes, or until the
    mixture thickens. The berries will
    break apart spontaneously, leaving a
    mildly chunky sauce.

3. Crush the berries with a fork or
    masher for a smoother sauce. Remove
    yourself from the sun. In six cups, add
    1/2 cup of yogurt and finish with
    sauce and toasted almonds.

INGREDIENTS

3 cups low-fat plain Greek yogurt

6 tablespoons sliced toasted almonds

STEPS FOR COOKING